Ask The Good Doctor:

The Detox Edition *REMIXED*

For a Healthy New You

IØ116665

By

DR. LAJOYCE BROOKSHIRE

Naturopath, Doctor of Naturopathic Ministry,
Master Herbalist. Licensed & Ordained Pastor

Renewing Your Mind Ink

Copyright 2019 © Dr. LaJoyce Brookshire

PUBLISHER'S NOTE:

Printed and bound in the United States of America. All rights reserved.

No part of this book may be reproduced or transmitted in any form or by any means, electronic or mechanical, including photocopying, recording, or by any information storage and retrieval system except by a reviewer who may quote brief passages in a review to be printed in a magazine, newspaper, or on the Web without permission in writing from the publisher.

Ordering Information: Quantity sales. Special discounts are available on quantity purchases by corporations, associations, and others. For details, contact the publisher at the address below.

Although the author and publisher have made every effort to ensure the accuracy and completeness of information contained in this book, we assume no responsibility for errors, inaccuracies, omissions, or any inconsistency herein.

ISBN: 978-1-58441-001-0

Renewing Your Mind Ink and Peace in the Storm Publishing, LLC. Visit our Website at www.peaceinthestormpublishing.com

ACKNOWLEDGEMENTS

Thank you for purchasing this book as it is my written commitment to ensure that you maintain, attain, and reclaim your Perfect Health. This **DETOX EDITION** *REMIXED* would not have been possible without the help of the following people in my Village and on my Team:

My Lord and Savior Jesus The Christ for shining His Light into my life and for giving me the Grace to allow His light to shine so men may see my good works.

My Husband Gus for being the best Royal Taste-Tester EVER, for putting-up with my incessant need to ensure we are healthy with this-and-that, the meals I create from scratch that I have dreamt-up or found in a magazine, and for praising the food hits and tolerating the misses. Who loves you Bay-ba!??

My Angel Baby for learning how to deliciously create Smoothies, shake the Eggnog, and beautifully plate a Nish-Nosh platter, thank you for drinking every new health drink -- no matter what it tastes like. I feel wonderful knowing you can go into the world with a solid health foundation. I love the little Brooke!

My Mommie Joana for giving me space to become the only Vegetarian in the household by keeping fresh fruit and veggies on hand and for encouraging my college roommates NOT to share food with me because I ate things they probably would not like to eat every day. Thank you for all you do! Love you!

Cindy Rodgers for giving the Persuasive Speech in 1979 at Kenwood Academy in Mrs. Stein's class about "Why You Should Become a Vegetarian" with diagrams. I was so persuaded by her speech that I changed my diet on the spot that day! Thank you, Cindy, for helping to set me on the Wellness path.

My Publisher Elissa Gabrielle CEO of Peace In The Storm Publishing, I thank you for seeing Renewing Your Mind INK as a viable outlet to share a few books with the world...all 1000 of them! I am ever so grateful for our partnership of which your mother would be proud. She would have loved to have seen the two of us making our marks in this world and in Publishing. For without her validating me in the Music Industry, who knows how long it would have taken for me – the new girl – to be accepted into the tightly knit circle of industry sisters. Let's get it...for Mike.

My SiriusXM Team – Karen Hunter, Program Director; Irvin Wright, Supervising Producer; Tremell McKenzie, Coordinating Producer; Michelle Joyce, The Digital Chick; Mo'sArts Mahogany & Wynter, Videography & Photography. Thank you all for taking an embryonic idea, stretching me to the max, and making it grow with your time and talents. You are all truly a Dream Team!

All of my Clients past, present, and future – Never, ever forget what you have learned as to why a Detox is essential in order to reap the benefit of maintaining Perfect Health…Pass it on.

<u>CREDITS:</u>

Cover Photo - Elijah (Farmer) Muhammad
for EM Photography

Make-Up - Lonai Mosely

Hair - Viviene Burgher

The Detox Edition *REMIXED*:
For a Healthy New You

It was January 1992, I was living my dream life in New York City in my dream career in the Entertainment Industry and I was happy and full of energy. My skin was radiant. I slept well and went to the bathroom like clockwork. I had no headaches or any other kind of aches or pains. In fact, I had never felt healthier. Then suddenly, after being under extreme stressful situations and the daily rigors of the New York City life, I started to experience just the opposite of all of the above and my body was screaming! This was about the time when my Holistic Doctor started encouraging me to do a Detox Program.

I was not convinced I needed a Detox back then until out of nowhere I got a bronchial infection that I had difficulty shaking. I was so ill that me, Miss Herbs and Pro-Organic Everything, resorted to taking two $80 rounds of antibiotics—and it still did not go away. The infection forced me to realize that I was not as healthy as I thought or looked. In line with my Naturopathic beliefs, I knew that my body had to be loaded with toxins to hold on to the infection so intensely.

What Exactly Is A Detox?

Most of Holistic Practitioners agree that a 'Detox' is a short-term intervention designed to eliminate toxins from the body promote health. A Detox is creating the perfect conditions to support our body in doing the job it was already made to do... "Detox."

Here are 10 Signs that your body is screaming for a Detox:

1. Constantly feel fatigued, stressed and overwhelmed

2. Experience headaches and/or lack of mental clarity

3. Often have skin breakouts and blemishes and/or a tired, dull and lack-luster complexion

4. Seem to pick up colds, flus, bugs and viruses easily and are often on medication

5. Digestion is troublesome, uncomfortable and irregular

6. Frequently slip into making less-healthy food choices often having fried foods, processed meat, dairy, gluten, processed foods, refined sugar or fast food

7. Frequently have coffee, soda, alcohol, cigarettes, drugs (prescription or otherwise)

8. Often exposed to common environmental toxins such as carbon emissions, cigarette smoke, herbicides, pesticides, artificial fragrances and household chemicals

9. Carrying excess body weight

10. Often feel emotionally unstable, depressed, unmotivated and lacking energy and enthusiasm for life

11. Have an allergic response to the change of seasons with scratching, sneezing, itching and wheezing.

If you can raise your hand to any of these symptoms, then a Detox is in order... NOW! A Detox is the opportunity to give your body a break and allow your own self-cleaning and self-healing processes to kick into gear. Our bodies are innately intelligent, and a period of cleansing is the perfect way to hit the reset button and start on a path to a healthier, happier, more vibrant you!

Here are just some of the benefits of a holistic, natural Detox:

- Prevention of Chronic Diseases

- Stronger Immunity

- Assistance in Losing Stagnant Weight

- Improved Quality of Life

- Increased Energy

- Radiant & Glowing Skin

- Bright, Clear Eyes

- Mental Clarity

- Balanced Emotions

- Improved Self-Confidence and Empowerment

- New Healthy Habits and Routines

- Improved Longevity

Kicking and screaming, I turned to the Detox program that was recommended. Remarkably, within 48 hours my ears that were clogged for weeks became unplugged. A day or two later my energy returned, my cough subsided, and I could breathe easier. I was surprised at how quickly the symptoms of the bronchial infection cleared up, but I was more shocked and a bit disgusted by the other effects the Detox had on me. Thick and varied colored mucus was escaping from every orifice of my body. My breath was foul. My armpits were funky. There was crusty stuff coming out of my ears and white mucus build-up was constantly in the corners of my eyes.

Still, I stuck with it, and after completing the 21-day program I felt like brand-new money. My body felt whistle-clean through and through. Complete strangers would tell me I had a 'glow'. It wasn't just my skin, it was my Spirit. The cleanse was incredibly powerful. The whites of my eyes were bright. My nails were pink and strong. My skin was supple. I enjoyed a deeper sleep. I no longer had cravings for salt or sugar or anything un-healthy. My bowel movements were five times a day, did not smell, and broke apart when flushed.

Although at first, I was reluctant to do the Detox, I now realize that it is a beautiful process, and I perform this rebirthing at the beginning of every season. I am pleased that you have decided to join me in this life-changing endeavor.

# # #

It is a new year or a new season, and you want a New You. I am sure you have made a vow to yourself, to your family, and to God that this is the year you will focus on being healthier. You love yourself and you want to stop abusing the temple that God has given to you. You also know that if you continue with your current behavior, disease is imminent.

There are certain poor habits that you would like to shake. To quote Fannie Lou Hamer, you are "Sick and tired of being sick and tired." You're tired of jumping up in the morning and pretending you got a good night's sleep and then drinking coffee, Red Bull, or 5-Hour Energy all day to stay awake. Deep down you may be terrified that you have inherited diseases from Mama and Daddy but have no idea what to do to ensure you don't get their ailments. Perhaps you are tired of the yo-yo effects of losing weight. Or you might be annoyed by the upset stomach that occurs after every meal and the indigestion that follows. I can imagine that you are also tired of taking laxatives to have bowel movements.

I hear you when you say you want a healthy lifestyle. I hear you when you complain that eating healthy foods cost too much. I hear you lament that your family and friends will not support your dietary changes and entice you with junk food and traditional food from your culture which have attributed to a long list of diseases in a long line of relatives.

I am here to help guide you to better health. I am here to help you to attain, maintain, and reclaim your Perfect Health. In this book, I offer a step-by-step approach to wellness. In 21 days, you will begin to see and feel a major difference in your body, which will encourage you to continue on this path toward attaining Perfect Health. By day 90 you will have instituted lifestyle changes that are effortless.

THE DETOXIFICATION PLAN

One of the MOST frequently asked questions is:

"Why do I need to Detox?"

The Answer is simple: We are assaulted daily with all types of toxins, from pollution to food additives. Our bodies should detoxify naturally—but unfortunately, this is not always the case. When our systems are overloaded, the natural cleansing process becomes sluggish. Some toxins—such as mercury and other heavy metals from seemingly harmless things like teeth fillings to tattoos and body piercing, in addition to the residues of prescription medications—are stubborn and do not necessarily leave the body on their own. This plan will help to breakdown toxins small enough into particles that can be excreted through the urine, bowel, and the skin.

WARNING When you engage in this Detox Plan and you are on medications for High Blood Pressure, Diabetes or anything else, your numbers will dramatically improve. You MUST monitor the numbers daily. For Example, when monitoring High Blood Pressure every day and your chart shows the numbers are normal for 10 days or more, then it is time to contact your doctor to advise that after implementing lifestyle changes your numbers have been normal for more than 10 days and it is time to talk about reducing the medication or coming off altogether.

IT IS VERY important to monitor your numbers daily! It is dangerous to take High Blood Pressure medications when your blood pressure is not high. More people die from taking High Blood Pressure medications when their blood pressure was not high. It is my hope that anyone taking High Blood Pressure medications owns a Blood Pressure Cuff and keep a record of your numbers each day.

To initiate the Detox Plan, then, we must give the body what it needs to eliminate waste by implementing the following steps:

Step 1: Drink Water

Water is crucial in the detox process. The Bible states, "Out of [your] belly shall flow rivers of living water" (John 7:38).

One purpose of a river is to transport debris. When we provide our body with water, the liquid in the body circulates blood and other fluids to cleanse toxins from the system. But this can only happen when we give the body enough water. When the body lacks proper hydration, the blood becomes stagnant and can clot. Blood and fluids collect poisons instead of eliminating them. The colon also becomes impacted with dry fecal matter and cannot do its job effectively. The bladder will then be forced to hold on to acrid urine increasing the chances of Bladder Cancer which is now the 4th most common cancer in men.

Improper hydration makes a clear case of Colon Cancer because fecal matter which cannot be moved out of the colon is trouble. Here is an analogy – How do you flush a toilet without enough water?

Have you ever taken note of a stagnant pool of water like a pond? It contains trash, dead insects, and a layer of dust particles, which combine to exude a foul odor. This is because the water is not flowing freely. This is similar to what happens inside the body when there is not enough water present to move around blood and fluids. (Note: this stagnation does not just occur in the colon, but all over the body).

How much is enough water? According to the book *Your Body's Many Cries for Water: You're Not Sick, You're Thirsty* by Dr. F. Batmanghelidj, -aka- Dr. Batman who says at the very least a person needs six to eight, 8-ounce glasses of water daily. You will know that your body is well hydrated when your urine is clear. This depends however on how much you weigh. Typically, the right ratio is to drink half of your weight in ounces daily. So, if you weigh 200lbs then your water intake should be 100 ounces per day. If this is still not producing clear urine then other factors are at play like prescription medications or vitamins which are not being utilized by the body properly and are being excreted. The answer...Drink more water until your Pee is clear!

A most common question asked is: What kind of water should I drink?

The Answer: During a Detox every effort should be made to drink filtered water, Alkaline water or Distilled water. I like Distilled water during this process because it melts the garbage in the body.

Many people believe that coffee, tea, soda, fruit juice and other beverages count toward the glasses of water needed. Many have been wrongly convinced that drinking Crystal Light, Gatorade, and Vitamin Water will satisfy thirst. In fact, none of this is true. When ingredients other than water are added, structurally and chemically a liquid is no longer water and becomes instead a water-based substance. The body does not recognize it as the kind of liquid it needs to cleanse itself. Instead, sugar, caffeine, and other ingredients hinder the cleansing process.

Caffeine is especially problematic. Americans love to "Run on Dunkin'" — and because of this, America is sick. Coffee is one of the most acidic agents on the planet. It takes 32 cups of water to flush out eight ounces of coffee (the same is true for soda). I know this seems like a lot of water and it is. That is how much water it will take to make it look like your body never had the coffee. (**Note:** Do not drink the water all at once. That can be dangerous.

Drink it throughout the day). Coffee contains Tannic Acid, which also contributes to dehydration and an acidic pH.

When striving for a body that is alkaline, the coffee is in opposition of the goal. Coffee is also a major dehydrating agent. Imagine a huge sponge rapidly soaking -up any water intended to hydrate the body. Just because something wet is close-by does not make it good for you.

I have heard every excuse under the sun about why water is not the primary beverage in a person's diet. The most discouraging one is, "I hate water." Someone who says this must also hate life. Not drinking enough water will eventually cause you to become sick and die. Water is the elixir of life. Every cell, every organ, every muscle needs water. In order for any metabolic reaction to happen in your body it needs to be hydrated. An example of a metabolic reaction is standing up and sitting down without pain. This is why Dr Batman says you're not sick you're thirsty. When you cannot stand up and sit down without pain you are dehydrated!

For the purpose of Detoxing, you should consume at least a 16- to 20-ounce glass of water every waking hour. Your first glass upon waking should be room temperature with the fresh-squeezed juice of half a lemon added.

During the Detox process, you are going to irrigate the toxins. Water will help to flush them out. You don't have to worry about overdosing on water, because most Americans are chronically dehydrated.

During the Detox process, it is important to make water the only beverage you drink. Herbal teas are also acceptable, but they do not replace the water requirement. Ensure that the herbal teas selected are truly herbal and not decaffeinated. The package should be labeled "naturally decaffeinated." Stay away from black tea, green tea, and white tea, as these contain caffeine. Yes, green tea is an excellent antioxidant, but during this process we are striving to make the body alkaline.

Step 2: Eliminate

During the Detox process and for the rest of your life, I encourage you to Pee and Poop On-Demand whenever and wherever nature calls. Unfortunately, many people so often feel inconvenienced by these natural acts. My clients have admitted to me that they urinate only twice a day and only have bowel movements at home. If you do not go to the bathroom when nature calls, you are essentially holding toxins in the body and working against the body's natural response to eliminate.

The goal should be to have clear urine, free of smell. The only urine of the day that should have a light color and mild odor is the first morning urine. Once you have begun drinking the prescribed amount of water, in a few days your urine should be clear.

This water will also facilitate smoother bowel movements. A healthy person will eliminate three to five times a day. The first reaction to this suggestion is usually, "That's not possible!" Not only are three to five eliminations possible, but for ultimate health it is absolutely necessary.

Due to our SAD (Standard American Diet), chronic constipation has become the norm.

Many mainstream doctors promote bowel movements once every couple of days as "normal." To that I say, find yourself a new doctor. Picture this: Imagine everything you ate yesterday on a platter. Now place it on the bathroom counter and turn the heat all the way up and close the door. (**Note:** I use the bathroom because it has close quarters and the door must be shut for the heat to be contained, similar to the colon — close quarters where heat is contained). Check on it in a couple of days. The rotten smell and sliminess of the food is what is left trapped in the body when there are not regular eliminations. This is the cause of most disease.

Your goal is for the poop to float or break apart when flushed. It should be the color of a baby's poop, light green to yellowish brown. You should also have a couple of eliminations before you leave home each morning. Once you begin drinking room-temperature water with lemon daily, you will have an immediate elimination upon rising.

Step 3: Eating Plan

During the Detox, consume fresh, organic, or farm-raised foods. Eat 5 to 7 servings of vegetables and 5 servings of fruit daily. I recognize that these foods tend to be more expensive. Yes, the stuff that has the dirt on it costs the most. However, I have heard from some people that although individual items are more costly, because they purchase less food overall — forgoing junk food — their total grocery bill is smaller. Remember, too, that you can pay now with money, or pay later with your health. In other words, spend your money on good food now, rather than on pharmaceutical drugs and medical visits later.

Every effort should be made to eat an Alkaline Diet which consists of at least 2 meals per day which are totally Alkaline. The foods which are Alkaline are mainly Vegetables and Fruit. It will be a bonus to challenge yourself to eat Alkaline foods for all of your meals by the last week of the Detox. Start slowly:

- Week 1 – Eat 1 Alkaline meal per day

- Week 2 – Eat 2 Alkaline meals per day

- Week 3 – Eat 3 Alkaline Meals per day

START OF THE DAY

- Upon rising in the morning, start your day with a 16- to 20-ounce glass of room-temperature water that contains the fresh-squeezed juice of half a lemon.

- Take supplements and vitamins as directed later in this chapter

- Make a Green Smoothie with Green Veggies and at least three fruits, water, and a powdered Multi-Vitamin/Multi-Mineral Supplement, and a MicroDaily Nutrient. (See Product Listing)

BREAKFAST

- Eat 3–5 servings of fresh fruit before 11 am.
- Eat individual fruit, fruit salad, Green Salad or fruit smoothies made with at least 3 servings of fruit (see Recipes). Do not combine melons with other fruits. Eat melons alone.
- If you feel the need to have a hot breakfast, Take Digestive Enzymes with breakfast, and

wait at least 60 minutes after eating fruit. When you eat fruit followed by hot food without waiting an hour, it creates excess acid in the digestive tract and hinders the elimination process.

LUNCH (EAT BETWEEN 11 AM AND 1 PM)

- 4–5 digestive enzymes followed by 20 ounces of water
- Raw green salad + protein

SNACKS

- Organic tortilla chips
- Hummus
- Granola
- Salsa
- Home-made Organic Popcorn in Coconut Oil or in Extra-Virgin Olive Oil w/Sea Salt
- Guacamole
- Organic yogurt
- Fruit (60 minutes before or after meals)
- Walnuts, pecans, almonds, sunflower seeds

DINNER (EAT BETWEEN 5 PM AND 7 PM)

- 4–5 digestive enzymes followed by 20 ounces of water.
- Raw green salad + protein + 2 servings cooked vegetables.
- As many vegetables as you desire to satisfy your appetite.

When your budget is tight, you may choose to purchase conventional foods, but try not to make sacrifices when it comes to certain fruits and vegetables. Non-organic produce items can contain up to 10 pesticides.

The Environmental Working Group (EWG) has specified 12 particularly problematic foods as its "Dirty Dozen." Avoid these and select your produce instead from the "CLEAN 15" — foods that expose you to fewer than two pesticides per day.

THE DIRTY DOZEN

1. Peaches
2. Apples
3. Sweet bell peppers
4. Celery
5. Nectarines

6. Strawberries
7. Cherries
8. Pears
9. Imported grapes
10. Spinach
11. Lettuce
12. Potatoes

THE CLEAN 15

1. Onions
2. Avocados
3. Sweet corn (frozen)
4. Pineapples
5. Mangoes
6. Asparagus
7. Sweet peas (frozen)
8. Kiwis
9. Bananas
10. Cabbage
11. Broccoli
12. Papayas
13. Eggplant
14. Watermelon
15. Sweet potatoes

While you're detoxing, there are certain foods that are best avoided altogether:

NO-NOs

Sweets

Artificial Sweeteners

Soda

Starch

Bread

Coffee

Purified Bottled water

Diet Soda

White Sugar

Beef

Deli Meat

Sparkling water

Margarine

Butter spreads

Pork

Packaged foods

White Rice

Sugar-free/dietetic foods

Decaf Teas

Iceberg Lettuce

Kool-Aid

Vitamin Water

Boost Drinks

Smoked meats

Non-organic yogurt

Popcorn

Ritz Crackers

Non-organic Vitamins

TV/Frozen Dinners

Canned Food

Gatorade

Energy Drinks

Fast Food

Pretzels

Non-organic dairy

Non-organic cereal

Peanuts

Non-Organic Juice

Non-Organic Salad Dressing

Microwavable meals of any kind   Alcoholic
                                    beverages

In addition, forgo use of the microwave altogether, as well as smoking.

To some, this list of NO-NOs may seem excessive, but keep in mind that the Detox program is for a short period of time. In order for it to be most effective, stop putting poisons into your body.

Step 4: Supplements

Detoxing is a rebuilding process. You are allowing your body to rest and restore itself by giving it what it needs. It takes five to seven times more nutrition to build and repair the body than it does to maintain it. Once the restoration phase is in motion, the quantities of supplementation can be decreased. You will be able to find the vitamins and supplements listed below online or at Whole Foods, Vitamin Shoppe, Vitacost.com,

Swanson.com, Amazon.com or at any good health food store.

MULTI-VITAMIN/MULTI-MINERAL

The vitamins I recommend are:

- Green Vibrance – by Vibrant Health

- VitaMineral Greens – by Health Force Nutritionals

- Amazing Grass – by Amazing Grass

- SuperFood -by Dr. Schulze American Botanical Pharmacy

I find these brands the most effective. When I finish with one, I rotate to the next. These products are super-foods containing energy-boosting and power cleansing chlorella, barley, blue-green algae, spirulina, and wheatgrass to name a few. If taken after 3 pm, it may impede your sleep.

Take 3 scoops of the multi-vitamin daily in Filtered or Distilled water with a mixture of half organic apple juice and half water. Drink three times a day before 3 pm. Alternatively, you could put 3 scoops of the powder in a fruit smoothie (see Recipes).

DIGESTIVE ENZYMES

DGL Chewable Original Formula is the digestive enzyme that I use. It is made by Enzymatic Therapy. Take 4–5 tablets of DGL with each home-cooked

meal. When you eat at a restaurant, take 5–6 tablets followed by 10-20 ounces of water.

COLON CLEANSE

It is important to keep all pathways of excretion open and flowing while intentionally Detoxing the body. When the Colon is blocked during this time, toxins will float all over the body. I like to see everyone take a colon cleanser for a couple of days ahead of the Parasite Cleanse to ensure everything is open and flowing.

For severe cases of constipation and after nothing else helps, I recommend a Colonic. I use Colonics as an emergency measure. I do not feel they should be used as maintenance. I once had to have one due to swallowing a chunk of an apple that I could feel which caused constipation. Another time I was under a great deal of family stress and was blocked as well. I needed a Colonic in both instances, and it worked.

The Colon is the second brain. Whatever may be of trouble to us emotionally and hard to process, the digestive process will also be slow to process. Hence, the elimination process will also be slow or

in my case during a really stressful and emotional period, come to a halt.

I like the following products:

- Intestinal Formula #1 – by Dr. Schulze American Botanical Pharmacy
- Super Bowel Pocket – by Russell Herbal Company

Follow the directions on the bottle of each. These supplements are effective only if you are properly hydrated, so follow it with 20 ounces of water. This should promote a prompt bowel movement the next morning between 5 and 7 am, if you eat between 5pm and 7pm.

PARASITE CLEANSE

The most common challenged concept is the protest on this issue: You are crazy Doc if you think I have Parasites!

Answer: We all have Parasites it is to what extent they bother you.

Dr. Frederick Douglas Burton is the Medical Doctor/Alternative Therapy Doctor with whom I studied who first educated me on Parasites. He went to the back woods of Tennessee to study with Chief Two Trees on the negative effects of Parasites remaining in the body. Dr. Burton passed his knowledge on to me. This is an issue of no debate with me. Everyone who comes to see me does this FIRST! I do not care what is wrong with you, let's move the buggers out of the way and get you feeling better immediately. There is a program called "Monsters Inside of Me" which proves that humans are the minority on the planet. As long as we are eating, drinking, breathing, and living there will be Parasites/Worms on the inside.

Imagine this: A person has died, and the body was not discovered for a few days only to find worms crawling out of every open body cavity. The worms did not crawl to the body, the worms crawled OUT of the body. Our insides are 98.6 degrees which makes it a nice warm and sticky host for the invaders to thrive. So, when we die, and are not tended to immediately the worms are doing their best to exit because there is no longer anything for them to feed on from us.

In my house, man, child, and beast start the Parasite cleansing process at every change of season around the 19th of December, March, June and September. If we are fastidious about De-

worming our animals, why then don't we deworm ourselves?

Here are some symptoms of Parasites being present:

• Seasonal Allergies – The Parasites are gestating (having more babies) at the change of every season which is why there is more dripping, sneezing, wheezing, and itching going on during this time than any other

• Asthma/Eczema – These two are the same disease, one being apparent inside the other apparent outside. Most people who have one also have the other or have had the two at some point in their lives.

• Diarrhea/Constipation

• Acne

• Foul Body Odor

• Dandruff

• Anemia

• Facial Swelling

• Itchy Ears, Eyes, Nose, Anus

• A traveling itch that cannot be satisfied

I recommend the following Parasite Cleanse/Deworming Products:

- ParaSmart – by Renew Life

- Scram – by HealthForce Nutritionals

- "Green" Black Walnut Wormwood Complex – by Now Foods

You can expect several physical changes during the parasite cleansing. You may experience itching, including anal itching. This is normal—the worms are on the run. Your body will be more "crusty" than usual. In the morning you may have mucus in the corners of your eyes. You may experience a foul taste in your mouth or bad breath. Do the following During the Parasite Cleanse:

- Brush teeth three times a day and floss daily – Parasites hide in the crevices of the mouth. Brush the tongue, cheeks, roof of mouth, and the crevice between the gums and lip line
- Use a Peroxide mouth wash mixed with Peppermint, Eucalyptus, Spearmint, or Tea Tree Oil
- Throw toothbrush away after the Parasite Cleanse is complete
- Take a bath or shower every night using an exfoliation cloth or sponge and a natural soap like Dr. Bronner's Castile Soap

- Use a clean bath towel every day. We get 3 million new skin cells daily and as the microscopic Parasites are coming through the skin which is the largest organ. Dead skin sloughing-off will be on the towel and it is wise to use a clean one daily.
- Clean the inside of your nose and ears with a cloth
- You will have a stronger body odor, dandruff, and increased earwax and/or flakiness
- Urine will be more acrid
- May see worms in your stool

These are positive indications that the body is excreting Parasites and worms. If you are squeamish about seeing worms in the toilet, then just wipe and flush. However, the single best way to monitor your health is to look at what is in the toilet and pay attention to the smell. Do the same for your family members. It is strongly recommended that while in the Parasite cleansing process that your sexual partner do the same or the two of you will pass the parasites back and forth.

Complementing the Detox Process

To enhance the expulsion process, every night during Detox cleanse, dry-brush the skin with a natural loofah (not plastic). Start at the feet and work your way toward the heart in a circular motion. This process stimulates the Lymphatic System. Dry-brushing daily for 30 days completely cleanses the Lymphatic System! This body system completely cleanses the entire body by removing the dirty fluid from the tissues. Consider the Lymph System as our internal oil change daily. When it is not operating at optimum capacity carrying out the waste the body will become sick.

Every other night take a soak in a tub of 1 cup of Epsom Salt, and 1 cup of Sea Salt. On another night use 1 cup of Baking Soda and 1 cup of Apple Cider Vinegar. This will assist in the elimination of toxins.

If a tub is not available, wet the body, and nightly make a different paste with the Apple Cider

Vinegar of the Epsom Salt, Sea Salt, Baking Soda and scrub it all over the body. It will feel so good and be like a spa treatment in the shower. Wash it off with the Castile Soap and moisturize with Coconut Oil, Extra Virgin Olive Oil, Shea or Cocoa Butter.

After the Epsom Salt Bath, perform Peroxide Therapy in your ears:

• Lying on one side of your body, pour $1/2$ cap of Peroxide into one ear well. Allow it to bubble for 5 to 15 minutes or until the bubbling subsides. Don't worry if the bubbles sometimes get hot, itch, and then cool; this is normal. Place tissue in the ear and turn your head to drain. Dry the ear well. Pinch off a piece of tissue large enough to plug the ear well to catch any remaining liquid. Repeat on the other side.

Many people have told me that this process makes them sleepy. To that I say, Good… go to sleep!

LIVER CLEANSE

The Liver is a major organ located in the upper right portion of the stomach which protects us from an abusive lifestyle. Its main function is to control the level of toxins in the body. It is critical that this organ operates properly. To promote maximum performance, I recommend cleansing it at least once per quarter especially if alcohol is consumed weekly.

There are many lifestyle habits which cause the Liver problems today. A missing Gallbladder, prescription drug residue, tattoo ink, frequent alcohol consumption, and processed foods do NOT leave the Liver on their own. It is up to you to maintain a healthy liver function.

A missing Gallbladder places a strain on the Liver like nothing else. The Gallbladder is a catch-basin for the Liver. Now with drive-by Gallbladder removals at the first sign of distress, the Liver is under siege. With every Gallbladder removal should be eating instructions so that the Liver will be safe. There should also be instructions on how to cleanse the Liver since its first line of defense is now M.I.A. But no... Allowing a patient to leave the hospital without a Gallbladder and no plan to protect the Liver is a most certain way to ensure the patient will return with a Liver problem.

I recommend the following:

• Complete Liver Cleanse – by Enzymatic Therapy

This is the perfect Liver Cleanse for a first timer. It is gentle and effective. Begin this two-week cleanse after the first seven days of your detox program and carry it through to the end.

For those with no Gallbladder, frequent drinkers, have tattoos, or take prescription drugs finish the Liver cleanse, wait 1 week and repeat.

- 5-Day Liver Cleanse – by Dr. Schulze American Botanical Pharmacy

Once you have done the Complete Liver Cleanse at least twice then move into this 5-Day Liver Cleanse. It is more intense and worth every moment.

If you have tattoos or no Gallbladder, after two cycles of Complete Liver Cleanse and one cycle of the 5-Day Liver Cleanse maintain the Liver daily with Milk Thistle capsules or tea daily.

WARNING: The Liver is the seat of the emotions. It is the place where anger is held in the body. Some say they are mean as a rattlesnake when they are cleansing the Liver and whatever comes up emotionally during this time comes out of the mouth…to that I say Bravo! It will serve your body well to say exactly what you feel when you feel it instead of swallowing your truth. You will feel liberated on many levels and that is the truth.

EVERYDAY MAINTENANCE SUPPLEMENTS

I want you to know that I will never recommend any products that I do not personally try myself. Every product recommended in this book have been tested by myself and my family. I am result oriented and NOT company loyal. First and foremost, I am seeking results from the best products. Some people who need extra support due to disease can benefit from the following products which I recommend:

- **RevitaBlu** – by Jeunesse Global

This product is a Stem Cell Nutrient. It is made from Sea Buckthorn Berry, Blue-Green Algae (from the pristine waters at Lake Klamath, Oregon), and Aloe Vera. Testimonies include one woman leaving behind 10 medications and no longer needing a knee or hip replacements.

After injuries and taking RevitaBlu, I have been able to run down steps again and that is priceless!

Try the product at:

www.DrLaJoyce.JeunesseGlobal.com

Or Email: Rsr@PermaHealth.com

- **Jamaica Moringa & Detox Pineapple Tea** – by Club BizSmart

This Moringa hails from the Red Dirt in Jamaica and it is what separates this product from the rest. Touted as being a Mighty Moringa Leaf due to minimal processing, the Testimonies include one man diagnosed with Mild Cognitive Impairment was able to avoid medication for Stage 1 of Alzheimer's. A 60-year-old woman lost 6 dress sizes in 6 weeks! And I have lost 12 pounds since taking the product in conjunction with Alkaline eating.

Try the product at:

www.JamaicaMoringa.com/DrBrookshire

Or Email: SVHood@msn.com

Micro Daily – by Engage Global

This product contains a high quotient of Micro-Nutrients which heal at the cellular level, break the blood-brain barrier, and repair oxidative stress which contributes to pre-mature ageing. It also contains natural free-radical and inflammation fighting agents. Most of us forget about Micro-nutrients and because they are depleted in the soil, we too are depleted. One woman reports that a Body Scan revealed her organs were more than 100 years old when she was 52 and after one month on Micro Daily the scan showed her organs were age appropriate!

I fell in love with this product and learned that it really does a job on Inflammation. I fell in a store injuring my knee and foot. I took Micro Daily Hydro Powder and capsules and two days later I was in high heels at a fashion show!

Try the product at:

www.DrBrookshire.Engage-Global.com

Or Call Engage Global:

801.655.4501

Reference Dr. Brookshire ID #156705

STEP 5: EXERCISE

Exercise is essential for our well-being—physical and emotional. In his "Golden Rules for Health,"

Naturopath Dr. Jack Ritchason tells us that we should exercise daily for the rest of our lives. You may complain that you are too tired or don't have the time. Did you know that exercising gives you more energy? Did you know that taking a brisk walk to the point of being breathless is considered exercise? As they say, Rome was not built in a day. Exercise is vitally important. Take it slow, increasing the number of repetitions and the amount of time you invest as you feel stronger.

Do 10 jumping jacks as soon as you get out of bed and before going to bed. This takes 30 seconds yet is a terrific Lymphatic System stimulator. Every couple of days, increase the number of jumping jacks you do by one. I torture myself with doing 100 of them, but I love the way I feel afterward.

EXERCISE STRATEGIES

- Park your car at the far end of a parking lot instead of at the door, then hustle up to the door fast enough to increase your heart rate.
- Take an extra spin inside a store with your cart. Caution: Don't spend extra just because you see extra stuff!
- Get off one train stop ahead and walk the rest of the way to your destination
- Make it a habit to take the stairs instead of escalators and elevators
- Enjoy a stroll after lunch or dinner
- Ride a bike rather than driving
- Buddy up with a friend and learn a new dancing skill — Zumba, African, Ballet, Ballroom, Hip-Hop
- Join a Gym
- Use the house as a Gym

Exercise is a habit we should never want to quit. Couple it with this Detox program, and you will see and feel amazing results. Weight loss is a bonus, and you do not have to replace real food with Special K or Slim-Fast Shakes to accomplish it. Exercise helps the weight to fall off naturally.

Step 6: Sleep

Question: What in the world does sleep have to do with a Detox program? Answer: Everything! The body only heals when you are sleeping. It is essential to get quality sleep at night. The moon is nature's healing agent. It restores and replenishes. The sun gives us energy. The healing cycle begins just before midnight at about 11:45 pm by restoring the Pineal Gland. In order to reap the benefits, you must be in REM (rapid eye movement) sleep at that hour. It takes two hours to establish REM sleep, so go to bed by 10pm. Get off that computer, turn off the TV, and

close the good book. Your body needs rest to be entirely well and to build a strong immune system.

Our immunity is weakened when we don't sleep as we should, or when we only sleep during odd hours. When we are sleep-deprived, we set ourselves on the vicious path of decaying health by flooding the body with all sorts of feel-better-for-the-moment foods and drinks.

Step 7: Prayer

The most essential part of this Detox period is

prayer. You will experience many energetic days when you will be thankful you have found these simple steps to enhance your life. Yet there may also be days when you want to quit because of cold- or flu-like symptoms. Please don't give up! Pray your way through. Don't look at what your body is going through as a problem; think of it as a promise of better health to come.

Those toxins do *not* want to leave. You may feel them going; as you do, say a little prayer for the strength to press on and a little prayer of thanksgiving that the toxins are exiting, leaving you healthier. You will find yourself really thankful after you have awakened from your restful nightly sleep. This alone is enough for you to forge ahead with the plan.

BEVERAGE RECIPES

A great companion to this book is my cookbook *Yes, You Are What You Eat: Recipes to Enhance Your Wellness Journey.* It is available exclusively through my website www.AskTheGoodDoctor.org

Here are the recipes promised to help you through this Detox period.

FRUIT H20

Here is the REAL Fruit H20! No additives or preservatives. This is for those who really are challenged with drinking water, this recipe for Fruit Water is a great way to drink up!

• In a large pitcher or jar, cut up fruit(s) of your choice into pieces about 1-inch square until there is a layer spread over the bottom of the container.

• Great fruit choices include strawberries, raspberries, watermelon, peaches, pears, and kiwi.

• Pour filtered water on top of the fruit and set the container in the fridge overnight. By morning, the water will have taken on the flavor of the fruit. This beverage makes a nice change for soda and juice junkies who feel they have to drink something flavored to drink.

FRUIT SMOOTHIE

• Peel, core, and cut fruit of your choice, fresh or frozen, into a blender

- You can start with a banana, and add at least 2 more types

- Then add $1/2$ cup organic Apple & Eve apple juice or 1 Micro Daily Hydro

- 1 of cup water

- 2–3 scoops of Green Vibrance or SuperFood or Amazing Grass or VitaMineral Green Multi-Vitamin powder of your choice

- 1 Organic Yogurt

- Blend all ingredients until smooth

#

You may complete this detox program once at the change of every season, or minimally at the beginning of the year and again at midyear. Congratulations for taking the plunge this year and beginning your Wellness Journey. By initiating a lifestyle change, you will experience the blessing of the best you ever as you stay in Perfect Health.

Please be in touch with me I would love hear your Health Praise Report!

Write Me:

Wellspring Holistic Center
c/o Dr. LaJoyce Brookshire
243 East Brown Street
East Stroudsburg, PA 18301

Contact Info:

Website: **www.AskTheGoodDoctor.org**
Email: **AskTheGoodDoctor@msn.com**
Twitter: AskTheGoodDoc
Instagram: AskTheGoodDoctor
FaceBook: Ask The Good Doctor
YouTube: Ask The Good Doctor LaJoyce

If you have any trouble obtaining one of the products recommended in this book. please feel free to contact me.

Available for:

• Individual Consultations in person or by phone
• Wellness Workshops – Churches, Organizations, Events
• Workplace Wellness Workshops
• Group Cooking Lessons
• Kitchen Warriors: 101
• Wellness Warrior Weekend Getaways